COOKING with QUINOA

25 RECIPES FOR THE WORLD'S HEALTHIEST SUPER FOOD

Jessica Simmons

Cooking with Quinoa:

25+ Recipes For The World's Super Food

Jessica Simmons

Copyright © 2014

All rights reserved. No part of this publication may be reproduced, distributed, or transmitted in any form or by any means, including photocopying, recording, or other electronic or mechanical methods, without the prior written permission of the publisher, except in the case of brief quotations embodied in critical reviews and certain other noncommercial uses permitted by copyright law. For permission, direct requests to the publisher, addressed "Attention: Permissions Coordinator," at the address below.

Distribution of this e-book without the prior permission of the author is illegal, and therefore punishable by law.

Disclaimer

Legal Notice: - The author and publisher of this book and the accompanying materials have used their best efforts in preparing the material. The author and publisher make no representation or warranties with respect to the accuracy, applicability, fitness or completeness of the contents of this book. The information contained in this book is strictly for educational purposes. Therefore, if you wish to apply ideas contained in this book, you are taking full responsibility for your actions.

The author and publisher disclaim any warranties (express or implied), merchantability, or fitness for any particular purpose. The author and publisher shall in no event be held liable to any party for any direct, indirect, punitive, special, incidental or other consequential damages arising directly or indirectly from any use of this material, which is provided "as is", and without warranties.

As always, the advice of a competent legal, tax, accounting or other professional should be sought. The author and publisher do not warrant the performance, effectiveness or applicability of any sites listed or linked to in this book. All links are for information purposes only and are not warranted for content, accuracy or any other implied or explicit purpose.

Letter From The Author

I just wanted to thank you for purchasing my book, "**Cooking With Quinoa: 25 Recipes For The World's Healthiest Super Food**". Quinoa is a super grain that more people are starting to incorporate in their everyday eating. Quinoa is not only good for you but taste great as well. I created this book to give you information about quinoa. I also wanted to show the many benefits of quinoa. This book gives many ways that this tasty grain can be incorporated into everyday cooking.

I personally use these recipes and can assure you that your family will love them. Once again thank you and I truly hope that you enjoy this recipe book and can bring these great and tasty recipes to your family's table.

Table of Contents

Table of Contents   5

Introduction   8

How Quinoa is Changing How the World Eats   9

5 Proven Benefits   9

Quinoa Helps Prevent Chronic Diseases and Cancers 9

Quinoa Prevents Nutritional Deficiencies   10

Quinoa and Allergies   10

What Is Quinoa?   11

Not a grain, a seed 11

Where did quinoa come from?   11

A Few Facts about Quinoa   11

Tips for Eating and Cooking Quinoa: 12

Types of Quinoa   13

Red Quinoa   13

White Quinoa 13

Black Quinoa 14

Which should you use? 14

Chinese Quinoa Recipes   15

Chinese Quinoa Rice   15

Tofu and Quinoa Stir Fry   16

Spring Onion Quinoa   17

Rising Dragon   18

Cold Chinese Chicken with Quinoa   19

Mediterranean Recipes with Quinoa   21

Mediterranean Harvest   21

Sunset Quinoa Salad   22

Greek Shrimp with Olives   23

Continental Recipes with Quinoa 26

Quinoa Pepper Gratin   26

Provençale Quinoa   27

 Almond and Chive Quinoa   29

Dijon Cake   30

Quinoa Baked Rounds   31

Indian Recipes with Quinoa   33

Upma   33

Mint Quinoa Side   34

Curried Quinoa with Raita   35

North American Quinoa Dishes   37

Artichoke and Quinoa Delight   37

The Flower and the Sword   38

Mushroom and Leek Quinoa 39

Sweet Bean Quinoa   40

Stuffed Squash   41

Japanese Style Quinoa   42

South American Recipes with Quinoa   45

Enchilada Bean Bake   45

Poblano Corn Quinoa   46

Roasted Chili Quinoa   47

Spicy Quinoa with Mole 49

Italian Recipes with Quinoa   51

Porcini Risotto   51

Sweet Potato Noodles with Chicken in Alfredo   52

Orchard Quinoa   53

Zucchini Pasta with Vegan Meatballs   54

Spinach Quinoa with Tomato and Garlic   56

Conclusion   58

Introduction

I want to thank you and congratulate you for buying the book, "Cooking with Quinoa: 25+ Recipes For The World's Super Food".

This book contains proven steps and strategies on how to start cooking with quinoa no matter what the recipe you are making or country the food is from!

Quinoa is changing the way the world eats. Whether you like Chinese, Mediterranean, Continental, Italian or Indian cuisine you will discover that many of the traditional recipes are using quinoa instead of rice or pasta. Not only does quinoa taste good, but also it is a super food that is scientifically proven to help lower your risk of chronic diseases and some cancers, while improving your nutrition and diet. If you want to get healthy, this is the book that will show you that you don't have to stop eating the dishes you love – you can just learn how to make them with quinoa!

How Quinoa is Changing How the World Eats

Many countries and cultures all over the world have taken to adapting their traditional recipes to include quinoa. As more and more become known about the health benefits of quinoa, you can see how it can not only improve your health – but it can play an important role in reducing risk for chronic diseases and some cancers.

Quinoa also plays an important role in creating gluten free and low glycemic index diets that deliver all the nutrition you need. It is easy to make and you can use it to replace rice, pasta and potatoes in almost all your recipes. You can even use quinoa flour to create a healthier meal no matter what the recipe!

5 Proven Benefits

1.   Quinoa provides an unusually high amount of protein. It has more protein than an equivalent serving of rice, wheat or other grains. The protein is very similar to that found in milk products, so it is easy to digest but doesn't have the associated lactase in milk that can cause problems.

2.   Quinoa provides one of the best sources of riboflavin, and calcium, you can find. This is important not just for your health; but if you are on a low GI diet, are gluten sensitive, lactose intolerant, vegetarian or vegan – these are common deficiencies. Riboflavin also plays a key role in helping keep your cognitive functioning high as you age.

3.   That bitter saponin coating doesn't just make for a good and natural laundry detergent; it is also an antiseptic that can promote healing of cuts and bruises.

4.   Looking for a low calorie, high protein and nutrient snack? Look no further than quinoa. ¼ cup of uncooked quinoa has only 172 calories.

5.   Quinoa is not a grain; it is a seed for a type of grain. That grain is not wheat. This makes it an ideal choice for those with celiac disease or who need to follow a gluten free diet.

Quinoa Helps Prevent Chronic Diseases and Cancers

There is a now a proven direct link between many chronic health conditions and consumption of meat based proteins. While many people are switching to leaner cuts of meat and avoiding the skin on poultry and fish, the push to switch to the leaner meats isn't the answer. In a new round of surveys done by the United Nations, the Food and Agricultural Organization paired with the National Cancer Institute to look at meat protein consumption to gain further insight into how consuming meat may be fuelling epidemics of chronic but avoidable diseases such as obesity, some cancers and Type 2 diabetes.

Quinoa Prevents Nutritional Deficiencies

One of the biggest criticisms you will hear about going switching to getting most of your protein from plant sources is that it will make you sick due to causing nutritional deficiencies. While there is some truth in the fact that there is a risk for some people to experience nutritional deficiencies while on eating a diet rich in plant protein, the real fact is that avoiding nutritional deficiencies is ridiculously easy. This is one of the reasons that quinoa has so much proven data behind it as a super food – it is a powerful source of protein that also carries important levels of vitamins and other nutrients that can become deficient in a plant based diet. With quinoa on hand, you won't have to worry.

Quinoa and Allergies

While quinoa does have a bitter coating called saponin, few people are known to be allergic to it. Quinoa does have high levels of purines and oxalates; if you are sensitive to either of those then you should not eat quinoa. While this is considered to be a "super food," eating too much of it can also cause problems. Always make sure to maintain a healthy, and balanced diet.

What Is Quinoa?

Quinoa is taking the world by storm as a "new" super food that promises to deliver a punch, without you having to lose anything in taste. Originally called "the mother seed" by the Incas, it has long been consumed as a staple of the South American diet. It is slightly sweet, nutritious, full of protein, full of good fats and nutrients and best of all – an ideal replacement for rices, flours and pastas for those with a gluten sensitivity or who need a low glycemic diet.

Not a grain, a seed

Quinoa is often mistakenly placed with grains in diet plans but it is not a grain at all. It is a seed for a grain. When consumed before germination, quinoa provides much more in nutrition and taste than its fully matured grain version can.

Where did quinoa come from?

Quinoa has an unusual history, not so much in how it came to be used as a food, but that it is one of the few times that American intervention in indigenous life had a positive side. Quinoa is native to the Andes Mountains; and is most common in the area of Peru. Since the time of the Incas, it had been a staple part of the diet of indigenous peoples.

When the Spanish invaded, they outlawed the farming and harvesting of Quinoa to try and force the people to adopt the more Westernized grains instead. Not only did the Spanish need the work force to focus on growing and raising grains, they also wanted to create an economy that was dependent on milling and imports. Quinoa was almost wiped off the face of the earth, but several areas were able to continue growing and using what has been traditionally referred to as "the mother seed."

In the 1980s, a group of Americans rediscovered quinoa and began to investigate its nutrition properties. Surprised to have discovered such a powerful and little known super food this led to a resurgence of harvesting and the introduction of quinoa to a much broader market. The Americans brought the seed to the Rocky Mountains in Colorado and began growing and selling it there, which led to interest in other harvests in Latin America.

A Few Facts about Quinoa

Here are a few facts about quinoa that may surprise you –

That bitter coating you will want to wash away is called "saponin" and is used as a laundry detergent in Latin America.

Scientists decided to genetically modify quinoa so it wouldn't have a bitter coating. It didn't work too well as the birds came and ate all of the seeds before they could be harvested. This is why you won't find GMO quinoa on the shelves. It is just plain and natural.

While quinoa comes from the Andes, over 200,000 lbs. are grown in the US each year. Quinoa needs altitude, but can use any mountain to grow on and thrive. In the US, you can find quinoa growing in the Rocky Mountains.

The higher quinoa is grown the sweeter it becomes. If you want sweet, find seeds that are marked as having been grown above 12,500 feet above sea level.

Tips for Eating and Cooking Quinoa:

There are more tips in this book to help you learn how to get the most out of eating and cooking quinoa but here are a few of the most common things to remember:

Always rinse the seeds well. Quinoa are "smart seeds" which means they have a protective bitter coating that is designed to make birds and other seed eating creatures avoid them. Soak the seeds and rub them together for the best result. You can tell when they have been rinsed thoroughly because there will no longer be soap like residue on the seeds and the water should run clear when drained.

Quinoa flour and flakes can be used instead of regular cereals and flours to create a truly gluten free baking kitchen.

A simple recipe substitution is to use quinoa whenever a recipe calls for brown rice. Brown rice can be hard for people with gluten or sugar sensitivities to handle.

You can pop quinoa seeds on the stove top in oil just like popcorn – add a little butter and salt and you now have a traditional Peruvian treat!

Types of Quinoa

There are over a 100 different types of quinoa available. Almost all quinoa comes from the Andes, and while there is a huge variety – you will most likely only encounter three.

Red

Black

White

Each of these main types of quinoa is used for different reasons in cooking, but all of them will deliver the same health benefits that you are looking for. Quinoa is not just available in seed form, but you can also find it as a flake and flour. You should consider replacing your breakfast cereal with quinoa flakes, using the flakes instead of a breadcrumb coating and replacing your regular flour in recipes with quinoa flour to get the most from this delicious and healthy food.

Why it's not considered a grain (although it sort of is)

It seems like splitting hairs when quinoa is declared to not be a grain, because it is a seed for a grain. In its seed form, quinoa does not have many of the aspects of other whole grains that can make them difficult for people to eat that may be gluten sensitive, have celiac disease or are looking to avoid starch. In its seed form, quinoa is packed with vital nutrients and provides a valuable source of plant protein that can help you keep going throughout your day.

Red Quinoa

Red quinoa has a rich color that makes it ideal for use with salads and other dishes were you need more variety than white. Many people who cook with red quinoa say that it holds it shape better than the white or black versions and has less of a tendency to become mushy. It is ideal for cold dishes because it does keep such a strong form.

White Quinoa

White quinoa is the most common to find and is sometimes called "ivory quinoa." It is inexpensive, easy to cook and can last for a long time uncooked if stored in an airtight container. White quinoa can be tenderer than the colored variety, which also means that it does not hold its shape as well. It is an ideal replacement for rices and pastas in a diet. The fact that it is similar in color to rice and pasta also helps even picky eaters be encouraged to try it. White quinoa is most often mistaken for a grain or pasta because it is so similar in behavior, texture and taste.

Black Quinoa

Black quinoa is "sweeter" than the other two and has a distinctive nutty flavor as well. It holds its shape as well as the red quinoa and its color too. It is a good choice for soups and cold salads. One thing you should know is that unlike black beans, the black of the quinoa won't seep out to color all the food it is mixed with.

Which should you use?

While quinoa does have a taste, it isn't overwhelming and the red, black or white styles can go well with any dish. The black is the most distinctive and works well when you need a sweet note added.

A fun mix to try is a little bit of each color so you can get a feel for the differences between them. It can also provide a surprisingly simple way to liven up a plate.

Chinese Quinoa Recipes

While quinoa originates from a much different part of the world, it adapts perfectly to Chinese recipes. Quinoa brings to these recipes an easy way to make them healthier, adding protein and fiber without sacrificing any of the flavors of these traditional dishes that you love.

Chinese Quinoa Rice

This really isn't a rice dish; the quinoa is used to replace the usual fried rice side with an equally flavorful option. With a touch of ginger it takes on an even more unique flair. With more protein and fiber than rice and offer, using quinoa with your Chinese meals instead of fried of boiled rice is a healthier alternative too!

You Will Need:

2 cups cooked quinoa

1 tbsp. coconut oil

2 eggs

3 cloves garlic

1 tbsp. fresh ginger

1 sweet onion

¾ cup peas

¾ cup carrots

3 scallions

2½ tbsp. soy sauce

¾ tsp. sesame oil

To Prepare:

Rinse the Quinoa with warm water and a dash of salt to remove the bitter outer coating.

Stir the quinoa while rinsing and use a fine mesh strainer. Shake the strainer to remove excess water before proceeding.

Bring water to a boil, add quinoa and simmer until all the liquid is absorbed.

Drain the excess liquid from the quinoa and fluff.

1. Chop the carrots into small cubes. Grate the ginger. Mince the garlic and chop both onions (but keep them separate).

2. Mix the sesame oil and soy sauce together in a small dish and set aside.

3. Brown onion in oil on stove top and then add the garlic with carrot cubes. Cook for 5 minutes while constantly stirring. Reduce the heat and let it simmer.

4. Add in all but the eggs and sauce/oil mix. Keep pinch of the scallions out for later too. Stir until all the liquid is absorbed and then push the mix to the sides to create an opening in the middle.

5. Whisk the eggs in a bowl and pour into the open middle in the saucepan and scramble. Mix the eggs with the rest of the pan items. Serve and top with the scallions kept back.

Tofu and Quinoa Stir Fry

One of the gifts of China to the rest of the world is their method of stir-frying. This provides a quick way to cook and combine ingredients without anything losing its flavor or flair. With quinoa, you get a fuller meal that everyone will enjoy.

You Will Need:

2 tsp. coconut oil

8 oz. extra-firm tofu

12 oz. mixed stir-fry vegetables

3 cloves of garlic

1 tbsp. ginger root

4 cups cooked quinoa

1/3 cup green onions

1/4 cup teriyaki sauce

Toasted sesame seeds

To Prepare:

Rinse the Quinoa with warm water and a dash of salt to remove the bitter outer coating.

Stir the quinoa while rinsing and use a fine mesh strainer. Shake the strainer to remove excess water before proceeding.

Bring water to a boil, add quinoa and simmer until all the liquid is absorbed.

Drain the excess liquid from the quinoa and fluff.

1. Cut the tofu into small cubes and brown the tofu in hot oil evenly. Remove and drain the tofu and place it aside.

2. Mince the garlic and ginger.

3. Use the same oil to stir fry the vegetables. Cooking them for 2 or 3 minutes while constantly stirring over a high heat.

4. Mix in the garlic and ginger to the vegetables and stir well. Add the tofu and quinoa, onions and spices and cook until warmed completely.

5. Remove and serve with a light topping of sesame seeds.

Spring Onion Quinoa

This is an easy and bright way to add a touch of the Orient to any meal. It can be served as a main dish or a side. It can also be made in advance and refrigerated as the perfect add-on for lunches or dinner throughout the week.

You Will Need:

1 tbsp. olive oil

1 cup quinoa

2 cups chicken broth

2 tbsp. low-sodium soy sauce

1 tbsp. ginger root

1 clove garlic

2 green onions

To Prepare:

Rinse the Quinoa with warm water and a dash of salt to remove the bitter outer coating.

Stir the quinoa while rinsing and use a fine mesh strainer. Shake the strainer to remove excess water before proceeding.

Bring water to a boil, add quinoa and simmer until all the liquid is absorbed.

Drain the excess liquid from the quinoa and fluff.

1. Mince the garlic and ginger.

2. Chop onions.

3. Heat the oil in a pan.

4. Toast the quinoa in the oil until brown for about 4 minutes.

5. Pour the broth in over the quinoa and add soy sauce with garlic and ginger. Boil and then reduce and simmer until all the liquid is absorbed.

6. Fluff and top with green onions before serving.

Rising Dragon

This brightly colored dish is a favorite for its surprising flavor. It can be made in advance and makes a perfect lunch or light meal!

You Will Need:

1 2/3 cups vegetable broth

1 cup red quinoa, uncooked

1/4 cup sliced almonds

2 tbsp. lemon juice

2 tsp. coconut oil

2 tsp. dark sesame oil

1/4 tsp. salt

3 green onions

2 tbsp. ginger, grated

To Prepare:

Rinse the Quinoa with warm water and a dash of salt to remove the bitter outer coating.

Stir the quinoa while rinsing and use a fine mesh strainer. Shake the strainer to remove excess water before proceeding.

Bring broth to a boil, add quinoa and simmer until all the liquid is absorbed.

Drain the excess liquid from the quinoa and fluff.

1. Add quinoa to a large bowl.

2. Mix in the remainder of the ingredients. Chill one hour before serving. Top with ginger.

Cold Chinese Chicken with Quinoa

Here is a quick dish you can make using pre-cooked chicken. You can also cook the quinoa in advance. If you want to add extra flavor, cook the quinoa in a ginger infused broth until the liquid is absorbed.

You Will Need:

½ cup quinoa, uncooked

Pre-cooked rotisserie chicken

2 tbsp. toasted sesame oil

2 tbsp. rice vinegar

1 tsp soy sauce

1 tsp agave syrup

1 small clove of garlic

2 celery stalks

2 scallions

¼ cup almond slices

To Prepare:

Rinse the Quinoa with warm water and a dash of salt to remove the bitter outer coating.

Stir the quinoa while rinsing and use a fine mesh strainer. Shake the strainer to remove excess water before proceeding.

Bring water to a boil, add quinoa and simmer until all the liquid is absorbed.

Drain the excess liquid from the quinoa and fluff.

1. Mince the garlic, celery and scallions but keep them separate.

2. Shred the chicken.

3. Combine the chicken with the oil, rice-vinegar, soy sauce, syrup and garlic in a bowl and mix to combine thoroughly.

4. Add in the cooked quinoa with onions and celery. Serve topped with almonds.

Mediterranean Recipes with Quinoa

Much of what you will find with the Mediterranean recipes is an emphasis on seafood and cool dishes. Quinoa is perfect as a simple side too.

Mediterranean Harvest

This is one of the best ways to use all the harvest you get from your garden. The bright and colorful salad also has a lot of room for personalization. Add a few cubes of ham or turkey to really change things up. If you want a vegetarian version, switch that to cubes of tofu.

You Will Need:

2 cups uncooked quinoa

3 cups fat-free, less-sodium chicken broth

2 tbsp. extra virgin olive oil

1 tsp. minced   mint

1 tsp. grated lemon rind

2 tsp.   lemon juice

1 tsp. sherry vinegar

½ tsp. sea salt

1 cup cherry tomatoes, quartered

1 cup thinly sliced radicchio

½ cup chopped yellow bell pepper

½ cup chopped cucumber

⅓ cup (about 1½ ounces) crumbled feta

3 tbsp. chopped pitted olives

1 tbsp. minced shallots

To Prepare:

Rinse the Quinoa with warm water and a dash of salt to remove the bitter outer coating.

Stir the quinoa while rinsing and use a fine mesh strainer. Shake the strainer to remove excess water before proceeding.

Bring broth to a boil, add quinoa and simmer until all the liquid is absorbed.

Drain the excess liquid from the quinoa and fluff.

1. In a large bowl combine the rest of the ingredients and the cooked quinoa and mix.

Sunset Quinoa Salad

Add in some blood-orange and a few other flavorful fruits to create a quinoa salad that is as bright and stunning as a sunset. This salad keeps well and can make an ideal lunch.

You Will Need:

¼ cup chopped green onions

2 tsp. grated blood-orange rind

1 tsp grated lemon rind

2 tbsp. blood-orange juice

1 tbsp. lemon juice

2 tsp. chopped cilantro

¼ tsp salt

¼ tsp. ground coriander

¼ tsp. ground cumin

¼ tsp. paprika

3 tbsp. extra-virgin olive oil

1 cup uncooked quinoa

1¾ cups water

½ tsp. salt

1 cup blood-orange sections

1 cup diced avocado

6 whole kumquats, seeded and sliced

2 medium cooked beets, wedged

To Prepare:

Rinse the Quinoa with warm water and a dash of salt to remove the bitter outer coating.

Stir the quinoa while rinsing and use a fine mesh strainer. Shake the strainer to remove excess water before proceeding.

Bring broth to a boil, add quinoa and simmer until all the liquid is absorbed.

Drain the excess liquid from the quinoa and fluff.

1. Mix the first 10 ingredients in a bowl. Slowly pour in the oil while mixing. When ingredients are completely combined, set them aside.

2. Combine quinoa, a pinch of salt, blood orange sections, avocado, and kumquats in a separate bowl. Pour in the dressing you made in step one. Serve on plates with a topping of beet wedges.

Greek Shrimp with Olives

This is a cool way to get all the protein you need in the hot months. The combination of the quinoa, olives and shrimps make a dish that is sure to surprise and delight.

You Will Need:

1/4 cup lime juice,

10 tsp. extra virgin olive oil

8 olives, sliced

1 tsp. cumin,

1/4 tsp. pepper

1/8 tsp. paprika

4 garlic cloves

24 shrimp

3/4 cup quinoa

1/2 cup onion

1 cup water

1/2 tsp. salt

1/2 tsp. honey

1 cup cherry tomatoes

1/2 cup canned chickpeas

1 ounce feta, crumbled

1/4 cup chopped cilantro

To Prepare:

Rinse the Quinoa with warm water and a dash of salt to remove the bitter outer coating.

Stir the quinoa while rinsing and use a fine mesh strainer. Shake the strainer to remove excess water before proceeding.

Bring broth to a boil, add quinoa and simmer until all the liquid is absorbed.

Drain the excess liquid from the quinoa and fluff.

1. Preheat grill to high heat.

2. Mix limejuice, oil and spices in a bowl.

3. Devein and clean the shrimp and then put the shrimp in the sauce bowl and let sit for ½ hour in the refrigerator.

3. Sauté onion and add quinoa and 2 cloves of garlic to the pan. Add a cup of water and bring to a boil before reducing the heat and simmering until all of the water is absorbed.

4. Add the pan of quinoa to the shrimp bowl and mix.

5. Take the shrimp out of the bowl and place on grill rack. Grill 4 minutes, turning once half way through.

6. Serve the quinoa as a bed for the shrimp on each plate topped with sliced olives.

Continental Recipes with Quinoa

These recipes are adapted from the Continental cuisine of France, Portugal, Germany and more. Here is a hint – if you have a favorite continental recipe that you like, replace the rice, pasta or potato with quinoa to make it a healthier choice. Quinoa can also be used instead of breadcrumbs too.

Quinoa Pepper Gratin

This is ideal when served with a simple green salad. The pepper adds just the right kick that your   salad will cool down.

You Will Need:

5 tsp. extra virgin olive oil

2 cups red onion

1 1/2 cups red pepper

1 pound cut yellow squash

1 tbsp. minced garlic

1/2 cup quinoa

1/2 cup basil,

1 1/2 tsp. thyme

3/4 tsp. salt,

1/2 tsp. pepper

1/2 cup reduced-fat milk

3 ounces shredded Gruyere cheese

3 large eggs

1 1/2 ounces baguette

1 large tomato

To Prepare:

Rinse the Quinoa with warm water and a dash of salt to remove the bitter outer coating.

Stir the quinoa while rinsing and use a fine mesh strainer. Shake the strainer to remove excess water before proceeding.

Bring water to a boil, add quinoa and simmer until all the liquid is absorbed.

Drain the excess liquid from the quinoa and fluff.

1. Sauté onion in oil until clear. Chop and add in the bell pepper and cook for an additional minute. Add in chopped squash and minced garlic and sauté altogether for another 4 minutes. Remove the vegetables to a bowl.

2. Mix the rest of the ingredients, including the quinoa with the vegetables in the bowl. Transfer the mix to a baking dish.

3. Tear up bread into tiny pieces and toast in oil on stove top in skillet. Remove and spoon toasted bread on top of mix in baking dish.

3. Bake at 375 until the topping it brown.

Provençale Quinoa

This dish makes an ideal midday meal. It is derived from a recipe common to the Provençale region and features lots of vegetables. Add in the quinoa and you have a restorative meal that will keep you going through the rest of the day.

You Will Need:

2 tsp. extra-virgin olive oil

1 garlic clove, minced

1 cup organic vegetable broth

1 cup water

1 cup uncooked quinoa

1 1/2 tsp. thyme

1/4 tsp. salt

2 tsp. olive oil,

2 cups leek

4 garlic cloves

2 1/2 cups fennel slices

1 3/4 cups carrot

1/2 tsp. fennel seeds

1/2 cup white wine

1 cup vegetable broth

4 tsp. thyme,

1 can chickpeas

1 tbsp. lemon juice

1/4 tsp. salt

1/4 tsp. pepper

1 small package spinach

To Prepare:

Rinse the Quinoa with warm water and a dash of salt to remove the bitter outer coating.

Stir the quinoa while rinsing and use a fine mesh strainer. Shake the strainer to remove excess water before proceeding.

Bring broth to a boil, add quinoa and simmer until all the liquid is absorbed.

Drain the excess liquid from the quinoa and fluff.

1. Sauté garlic until tender in oil. Add broth, quinoa and simmer until all of the broth is absorbed. Cover and let sit.

2. Cook the rest of the ingredients together in a Dutch oven on medium until the chickpeas are tender. Remove and let cool. Serve as a topping to the quinoa mix in bowls.

Almond and Chive Quinoa

Almonds have a unique flavor that is strong and can stand up to meats and hardy fish steaks. With quinoa added in, you have the perfect side dish.

You Will Need:

1 cup uncooked quinoa

2 tsp. extra-virgin olive oil

2 tbsp. finely chopped shallots

1 tbsp. minced garlic

1 1/4 cups chicken broth

1/4 tsp. salt

1/4 cup almonds

1 tbsp. extra-virgin olive oil

1/4 cup chopped parsley

2 tbsp. chopped chives

1/4 tsp. pepper

To Prepare:

Rinse the Quinoa with warm water and a dash of salt to remove the bitter outer coating.

Stir the quinoa while rinsing and use a fine mesh strainer. Shake the strainer to remove excess water before proceeding.

Bring water to a boil, add quinoa and simmer until all the liquid is absorbed.

Drain the excess liquid from the quinoa and fluff.

1. Sauté shallots in oil on stovetop. Add minced garlic and heat through. Add quinoa and stir to heat. Add in the broth and salt, bring to a boil and then reduce and simmer until all of the liquid is absorbed.

2. In a separate pan, brown the almonds in oil. Then add the nuts with seasonings to the cooked quinoa.

Dijon Cake

This spicy treat from the coast that features fresh crab with the flavor of Dijon. It makes for a wonderful lunch or dinner entrée.

You Will Need:

4 cups vegetable broth

1/2 cup quinoa

1/2 tsp. black pepper

1/2 tsp. paprika

1/4 tsp. ground red pepper

1/4 cup Greek yogurt

1/4 cup mayonnaise

1/4 cup sweet pickles

1 tsp. Dijon

8 oz. crabmeat

1/4 cup red bell pepper

1/4 cup celery

1/4 cup green onions

1/2 tsp. salt

1 large egg

2 tbsp. coconut oil

To Prepare:

Rinse the Quinoa with warm water and a dash of salt to remove the bitter outer coating.

Stir the quinoa while rinsing and use a fine mesh strainer. Shake the strainer to remove excess water before proceeding.

Bring broth to a boil, add quinoa and simmer until all the liquid is absorbed.

Drain the excess liquid from the quinoa and fluff.

1. Chop the peppers, celery, onions and pickles (but keep all separate).

2. Mix everything together in a bowl. Use a large spoon to scoop out the mixture and drop the mix on a plate. Press the drops down to form patties. Allow the patties to set for 1 hour in the refrigerator.

3. Transfer the patties to a baking dish. Brush the tops with the oil. Place in the broiler and cook until each side is brown (turning once during the cook time).

Quinoa Baked Rounds

These are fun and easy. They create small baked "meatballs" that can be served as an appetizer or make a great choice as an add on to pasta.

You Will Need:

1/2 cup quinoa

1 lb. ground pork

1/2 cup shallot

4 garlic cloves

2 eggs

1/2 tsp. black pepper

1/2 tsp. cayenne pepper

1/2 tsp. paprika

1/2 tsp. oregano

1/2 tsp. parsley

1/4 tsp. ground cinnamon

To Prepare:

Rinse the Quinoa with warm water and a dash of salt to remove the bitter outer coating.

Stir the quinoa while rinsing and use a fine mesh strainer. Shake the strainer to remove excess water before proceeding.

Bring water to a boil, add quinoa and simmer until all the liquid is absorbed.

Drain the excess liquid from the quinoa and fluff.

1. Preheat the oven to 450. Smash the garlic.

2. Mix all of the ingredients in a bowl including the quinoa (once it has cooled).

3. Shape the mix into tiny meatballs and space evenly on a baking sheet.

4. Bake at 450 until brown and the centers are cooked.

Indian Recipes with Quinoa

Indian recipes are ideal for use with quinoa instead of rice. It can make them heartier, and gluten free!

Upma

Upma is a very traditional dish from India that is given a new life with the addition of quinoa. This is flavorful, but not as spicy as some of the curries.

You Will Need:

1 tbsp. ghee

¼ tsp. cumin

3-green chilies

1 onion

3 pieces peeled ginger root

¼ tsp.

½ cup cubed carrots

½ cup peas

2 cups quinoa, red or white

Fresh cilantro

To Prepare:

Rinse the Quinoa with warm water and a dash of salt to remove the bitter outer coating.

Stir the quinoa while rinsing and use a fine mesh strainer. Shake the strainer to remove excess water before proceeding.

1. Sauté the cumin, chilies, onion and ginger in the ghee until the onions are soft and clear.

2. Stir in turmeric, peas and carrots.

3. Stir in the rinsed, raw quinoa. Add the water and bring to a boil.

Cover and reduce the heat to a simmer. Simmer until the all the liquid is absorbed by the quinoa.

Mint Quinoa Side

This recipe can provide you with the perfect side dish to liven up any entrée. It also makes for an ideal low calorie snack salad that can pack a punch to keep your going.

You Will Need:

1 3/4 cups quinoa

2 tbsp. coconut oil

3 tbsp. shallots

2 cups water

1/3 cup dry white cooking wine

1/2 tsp. salt

3 tbsp. lemon juice

1/4 tsp. black pepper

1/4 cup mint

1/4 cup parsley

To Prepare:

Rinse the Quinoa with warm water and a dash of salt to remove the bitter outer coating.

Stir the quinoa while rinsing and use a fine mesh strainer. Shake the strainer to remove excess water before proceeding.

Bring water to a boil, add quinoa and simmer until all the liquid is absorbed.

Drain the excess liquid from the quinoa and fluff.

1. Chop the shallots and then sauté them in the cooking wine until soft.

2. Add quinoa and bring to boil. Reduce heat and simmer until liquid is

absorbed. Remove from stove and let cool.

3. In a large bowl, combine the remainder of the ingredients and then mix in the shallots and quinoa. Serve with a mint garnish.

2. Combine the remaining ingredients together in a large bowl with the cooled quinoa and serve.

Curried Quinoa with Raita

Curry is nice, but for some it can be too much. This is what makes this recipe such a success. It provides a balance to the curry flavor through cucumber and mint raita. This is a great way to expand the taste of your table. This recipe makes 6 servings.

You Will Need:

1 tsp. extra virgin olive oil

2 tsp. curry

1 garlic clove

1 cup quinoa

2 cups water

3/4 tsp. salt

1 diced mango

1/2 cup diced celery

1/4 cup green onions

3 tbsp. cilantro

3 tbsp. currants

1/4 cup cucumber

2 tsp. mint

1 carton plain yogurt

1 package spinach

To Prepare:

Rinse the Quinoa with warm water and a dash of salt to remove the bitter outer coating.

Stir the quinoa while rinsing and use a fine mesh strainer. Shake the strainer to remove excess water before proceeding.

Bring water to a boil, add quinoa and simmer until all the liquid is absorbed.

Drain the excess liquid from the quinoa and fluff.

1. Cook oil and curry in oil for about 1 minute. Add in the water and quinoa and bring all to a boil. Reduce heat and simmer until liquid is absorbed.

2. Dice mango and celery and add to quinoa along with onions, cilantro and currants. Mix together well.

3. In a separate bowl, mix the cucumber with mint and yogurt to make the raita. Put the spinach on each plate, then the quinoa mixture and top with the raita mix.

North American Quinoa Dishes

Here are just a few of the amazing recipes you can discover with quinoa as a featured ingredient. Try a few or try them all, and then experiment to create your own. One of the wonderful things about quinoa is that it is liked by many; even kids tend to enjoy it. No one has to know if you are switching to quinoa for health or diet reasons, they just have to know that it tastes good.

Artichoke and Quinoa Delight

This delightful and light spring salad is perfect for bringing in the season. The artichoke adds a rich flavor and texture, while the parsley provides a unique note.

You Will Need:

1 tbsp. olive oil

1 cup chopped spring or sweet onion

1/2 tsp. chopped thyme

1 (9-ounce) package frozen artichoke hearts, thawed

1 cup fat-free, lower-sodium chicken broth

1/2 cup uncooked quinoa

1 cup chopped parsley

5 tsp. grated lemon rind

1 1/2 tbsp. lemon juice

1/4 tsp. salt

To Prepare:

Rinse the Quinoa with warm water and a dash of salt to remove the bitter outer coating.

Stir the quinoa while rinsing and use a fine mesh strainer. Shake the strainer to remove excess water before proceeding.

1. Bring oil to a boil and add onions and thyme and cook until onion is soft. Add in artichokes and sauté.

2. Add broth and quinoa to the pan and cover. Simmer until all the liquid is gone.

2. Let all cool and then stir in the remaining ingredients until mixed well. Serve with salad.

The Flower and the Sword

Apricot and onion may sound like an unusual combination but the sweet and the sharp tastes provided in this salad will be sure to win fans. You can serve it as a side, or you can serve it as a light meal by itself.

You Will Need:

1 cup water

1/2 cup quinoa

3/4 cup parsley leaves

1/2 cup celery

1/2 cup green onions

1/2 cup apricots

3 tbsp. lemon juice

1 tbsp. olive oil

1 tbsp. honey

1/4 tsp. salt

1/4 tsp. black pepper

1/4 cup pumpkin seeds

To Prepare:

Rinse the Quinoa with warm water and a dash of salt to remove the bitter outer coating.

Stir the quinoa while rinsing and use a fine mesh strainer. Shake the strainer to remove excess water before proceeding.

Bring broth, parsley, apricots and celery to a boil, add quinoa and simmer until all the liquid is absorbed.

Drain the excess liquid from the quinoa and fluff.

1. Mix lemon juice, olive oil, honey, salt, and black pepper into cooled quinoa.

Mushroom and Leek Quinoa

This recipe brings out the super food nature of quinoa by combining it with shiitake mushrooms and leeks to create a protein power punch that is surprisingly light and flavorful.

You Will Need:

2 cups vegetable broth

1 cup water

1/2 tsp. salt,

1 1/2 cups quinoa

3 tbsp. parsley

1 tbsp. olive oil,

1/4 tsp. pepper

3 cups leeks

4 cups shiitake mushroom caps

1 1/2 cups red pepper

1/4 cup dry white wine

1/2 cup walnuts

To Prepare:

Rinse the Quinoa with warm water and a dash of salt to remove the bitter outer coating.

Stir the quinoa while rinsing and use a fine mesh strainer. Shake the strainer to remove excess water before proceeding.

Bring broth, parsley, oil and pepper to a boil, add quinoa and simmer until all the liquid is absorbed.

Drain the excess liquid from the quinoa and fluff.

1. Sauté leeks in oil until they wilt. Then stir in wine, mushrooms and pepper and cook until the mushrooms and pepper are soft.

2. Season quinoa mix with salt and pepper to taste and serve in bowls, topped with mushrooms and pepper mix with walnuts.

Sweet Bean Quinoa

Black beans are definitely a power food, but the surprising combination of a basil and lemon dressing balance out their taste and make for a refreshing salad that can be served with a meal, or as the main

You Will Need:

1 1/2 cups uncooked quinoa

3 cups vegetable broth

1 package tofu, cubed

3 tbsp. olive oil

1 1/4 tsp. salt

1 cup chopped basil

3 tbsp. lemon juice

2 tbsp. Dijon mustard

1 tsp. sugar

2 tsp. grated lemon rind

1/2 tsp. black pepper

3 garlic cloves, minced

1 (10-ounce) package frozen baby lima beans

4 cups chopped tomato (about 3-medium)

1/2 cup sliced green onions

1/2 cup chopped carrot

1 (15-ounce) can black beans, rinsed and drained

To Prepare:

Rinse the Quinoa with warm water and a dash of salt to remove the bitter outer coating.

Stir the quinoa while rinsing and use a fine mesh strainer. Shake the strainer to remove excess water before proceeding.

Bring broth to a boil, add quinoa and simmer until all the liquid is absorbed.

Drain the excess liquid from the quinoa and fluff.

1. Sauté tofu on high heat in skillet with a pinch of salt until the tofu is lightly browned on both sides.

2. Mix oil, salt, basil and spices (including garlic) in bowl and blend in quinoa.

3. Cook beans separately and then add all ingredients and mixes together. Refrigerate until chilled and serve.

Stuffed Squash

One of the nicest things about this recipe is that you can make it in advance. It is also easy to carry for a picnic or a lunch since each squash acts as its own container.

You Will Need:

4 golden squashes

Cooking spray

2 (4-ounce) links hot turkey Italian sausage

1/2 cup finely chopped carrot

1/2 cup finely chopped onion

2 garlic cloves, minced

1/2 cup water

2 cups cooked quinoa

2 tbsp. chopped parsley

1/2 tsp. chopped thyme

1/4 tsp.   salt

1/4 tsp. black pepper

3/4 cup (3 ounces) Monterey Jack cheese

To Prepare:

Rinse the Quinoa with warm water and a dash of salt to remove the bitter
outer coating.

Stir the quinoa while rinsing and use a fine mesh strainer. Shake the strainer
to remove excess water before proceeding.

Bring broth to a boil, add quinoa and simmer until all the liquid is absorbed.

Drain the excess liquid from the quinoa and fluff.

1. Slice the top of the squash up, seed the squash and set the
squashes together in a dish of water. There should only be about 1
inch of water total in the dish. Put the dish in a microwave and cook on
high for 15 minutes.

2. Remove the sausage meat from the skins and sauté until brown.
Spoon out the sausage and then add a ½ cup of water and bring to boil
with the carrots, garlic and chopped onion in the drippings. Reduce
heat, cover and simmer until the carrots can be cut with a fork.

4. Add the vegetable mix with the quinoa and sausage. Fill the
squashes with the mix and top with cheese. Bake for 20 minutes at
350.

Japanese Style Quinoa

This is a fun dish that uses the Japanese liquor, Sake, for flavor – and as a quick way to cure the salmon.

You Will Need:

1 salmon fillet

1 tsp. salt

2 tsp. sugar

1 1/2 cups sake

1/2 tsp. chili paste

2 garlic cloves, minced

1 cup quinoa

1 tsp. butter

1 1/2 tsp. olive oil

1/2 cup finely chopped red bell pepper

1/2 cup finely chopped carrot

1/4 cup finely chopped onion

1 cup water

1/2 cup orange juice

1/4 tsp. salt

1 tbsp. chopped parsley

To Prepare:

Rinse the Quinoa with warm water and a dash of salt to remove the bitter outer coating.

Stir the quinoa while rinsing and use a fine mesh strainer. Shake the strainer to remove excess water before proceeding.

Bring broth to a boil, add quinoa and simmer until all the liquid is absorbed.

Drain the excess liquid from the quinoa and fluff.

1. Prepare salmon by rubbing salt and sugar over both sides of the skin. Place in refrigerator, covered in plastic for several hours to chill. Remove the salmon and rinse. Put sake, sugar, chili and garlic in plastic bag, seal salmon inside and put back in refrigerator to marinate. Make sure you turn it once.

2. Melt butter in pan and then sauté pepper, carrots and onions until the onion is clear and tender.

3. Add in a cup of water, sake, juice to the pan and bring to boil. Add one pinch of salt and the quinoa. Boil and stir for about a minute, then reduce heat and simmer while covered until all the liquid is absorbed by the quinoa.

4. Take the salmon from the marinade bag. Reduce the marinade in a small pan on the stove and then brush the salmon on both sides with the reduction.

5. Pan sear both sides of salmon. Baste with marinade and then bake at 450 until fish flakes. Serve on top of bed of quinoa.

South American Recipes with Quinoa

South of the border you began to come close to the traditional use of quinoa in recipes. It is a brilliant way to add protein and fiber to any Latin American style meal. Here is another hint – if you are making your own tortillas, use quinoa flour instead of corn or wheat flour for a gluten free option.

Enchilada Bean Bake

One of the most traditional and best loved of all Mexican dishes, enchiladas are also easy to make. With quinoa and black beans as the foundation, this meal becomes a powerhouse of nutrition.

You Will Need:

1 cup quinoa

2 cups water

1 tbsp. olive oil

1-onion

3 cloves garlic

1 Jalapeño

1 Red pepper

1 Yellow pepper

1 cup corn

1 tbsp. lime juice

1 tsp. ground cumin

1 tbsp. chili powder

1/3 cup cilantro

2 cans black beans

2 cups red enchilada sauce

2 cups shredded Mexican cheese

To Prepare:

Rinse the Quinoa with warm water and a dash of salt to remove the bitter outer coating.

Stir the quinoa while rinsing and use a fine mesh strainer. Shake the strainer to remove excess water before proceeding.

Bring water to a boil, add quinoa and simmer until all the liquid is absorbed.

Drain the excess liquid from the quinoa and fluff.

1. Chop, seed and dice peppers and onions.

2. Turn oven on to 350 to heat.

3. Sauté onions and garlic with jalapeno in oil until soft. Mix in the rest of the peppers and corn and sauté together for 5 minutes.

4. Add limejuice and all seasoning. Stir thoroughly to mix in pan. Remove from heat.

5. Mix the quinoa with the drained and mixed beans in a large bowl. Add in the vegetables. Pour in the sauce and stir. Finally, add the cheese and stir in completely.

6. Pour the mix in a baking dish and put it in the oven, covered, for 20 minutes. Remove the foil, top with cheese and bake until cheese melts and browns.

Poblano Corn Quinoa

This tomato is stuffed with all sorts of goodness, including quinoa. Add a touch of limejuice to bring it all alive. This can be served as an appetizer, side or the main dish.

You Will Need:

2 Poblano chilies

2 cups corn

1 cup onion

1 tbsp. oregano

1 tbsp. olive oil

1 tbsp. lime juice

1 tsp. salt

3/4 tsp. cumin

1/4 tsp. black pepper

6 tomatoes

1 cup uncooked quinoa

2 cups water

4 oz. Colby cheese

To Prepare:

Rinse the Quinoa with warm water and a dash of salt to remove the bitter outer coating.

Stir the quinoa while rinsing and use a fine mesh strainer. Shake the strainer to remove excess water before proceeding.

Bring water to a boil, add quinoa and simmer until all the liquid is absorbed.

Drain the excess liquid from the quinoa and fluff.

1. Seed the chilies and blacken them in the broiler. Remove the chilies from the baking sheet and let them sit in a closed paper bag to remove excess oil. Remove the chilies from the oil and chop finely.

2. Broil onion and corn until tender. Chop and add with chilies.

3. Add all but tomatoes and quinoa to the mix.

4. Remove the top from the tomatoes and the pulp. Dry the inside of the tomato with a paper towel and lightly salt.

5. Add quinoa to the other ingredients and mix well.

6. Pack the tomatoes with a complete mix and top with cheese. Broil until cheese begins to bubble and turn brown.

Roasted Chili Quinoa

This is a vegetarian chili featuring quinoa that is sure to blast away the cold. It also is chocked full of protein, spicy flavors and everything you need to make a full meal. Serve it for lunch or dinner with a side salad and you have an easy to make meal that is sure to be a hit. This recipe makes 4 servings.

You Will Need:

2-red bell peppers

2-Poblano chilies

4 tsp. extra virgin olive oil

3 cups zucchini

1 1/2 cups onion

4 garlic cloves

1 tbsp. chili-powder

1 tsp. cumin

1/2 tsp. paprika

1/2 cup water

1/3 cup quinoa

1/4 tsp. salt

1 can diced tomatoes

1 can pinto beans

1 cup vegetable juice

To Prepare:

Rinse the Quinoa with warm water and a dash of salt to remove the bitter outer coating.

Stir the quinoa while rinsing and use a fine mesh strainer. Shake the strainer to remove excess water before proceeding.

Bring water to a boil, add quinoa and simmer until all the liquid is absorbed.

Drain the excess liquid from the quinoa and fluff.

1. Cut peppers and chilies in half, seed and clean. Place halves on a

baking sheet. Broil until blackened. Remove the peppers and put them in a paper bag. Let stand for about 10 minutes so the bag can absorb the excess juices. Remove the peppers and chop coarsely.

2. Coat the bottom of a Dutch oven with oil and heat the oven. Chop and then sauté the zucchini, onion, and garlic. Stir in spices and cook for an additional 30 seconds. Add the chopped peppers, 1/2 cup water, and the rest of the ingredients (including the quinoa). Reduce heat and simmer until the quinoa is tender but not mushy.

Spicy Quinoa with Mole

This is a great salad to make in advance. It keeps well. Just make the salad and the quinoa in two separate containers and combine them right before serving. This recipe makes 6 servings.

You Will Need:

1 tsp. orange rind

3/4 tsp. cocoa

1/2 tsp. cumin

1/2 tsp. cinnamon

2 tbsp. orange juice

1 1/2 tbsp. red-wine vinegar

1 tbsp. adobo sauce

2 tbsp. extra virgin olive oil

3 cups quinoa

6 cups water

1/2 cup toasted pepitas

1/4 cup chopped cilantro

1/2 tsp. salt

2 green onions

1 jalapeño pepper,

1 can black beans

4 cups baby spinach

To Prepare:

Rinse the Quinoa with warm water and a dash of salt to remove the bitter outer coating.

Stir the quinoa while rinsing and use a fine mesh strainer. Shake the strainer to remove excess water before proceeding.

Bring water to a boil, add quinoa and simmer until all the liquid is absorbed.

Drain the excess liquid from the quinoa and fluff.

1. Combine orange rind, cocoa, juice, vinegar and spices in small bowl – slowly add the oil and mix well.

2. Add in the quinoa and remainder of the ingredients. Toss well and serve over spinach.

Italian Recipes with Quinoa

These are some of the most flavorful Italian recipes adapted to use quinoa. They were chosen because they not only demonstrate how to use quinoa in place of traditional Italian ingredients, but the added instructions for how to make a vegetable pasta for gluten free dishes is something everyone should learn.

Porcini Risotto

The rich flavor and texture of the porcini mushroom is what provides the perfect capping taste to this dish. You can serve it over risotto, or spiralize zucchini for a gluten free dish.

You Will Need:

1 cup quinoa

2 oz. dried porcini

2 cups water

1 cup fresh mushrooms

1 bunch asparagus

3 cups spinach

1 shallot

2 garlic cloves

Salt and pepper

Extra virgin olive oil

Vegetable broth

To Prepare:

Rinse the Quinoa with warm water and a dash of salt to remove the bitter outer coating.

Stir the quinoa while rinsing and use a fine mesh strainer. Shake the strainer to remove excess water before proceeding.

Bring water to a boil, add quinoa and simmer until all the liquid is absorbed.

Drain the excess liquid from the quinoa and fluff.

1. Boil the mushrooms until they are cooked through, about 20 minutes. Drain the mushrooms.

2. Chop the garlic, shallots and mushrooms. Sauté them together until the onions are tender. Add asparagus and sauté until asparagus is soft. Add salt and pepper, a light dash each.

3. Add cooked quinoa and spinach. Sauté until spinach wilts and then mix in the vegetable broth, cover, reduce heat and simmer. Simmer until the liquid thickens to the preferred consistency.

4. Serve with grated cheese topped with pepper flakes (sparingly).

Sweet Potato Noodles with Chicken in Alfredo

This is a very rich and filling entrée. If you want to make the whole dish vegan substitute tofu for the chicken.

You Will Need:

For Alfredo:

1/2 cup raw cashews

2-cloves of garlic

1/4 cup yeast

1/2 cup quinoa

1 cup almond milk

2 tsp. soy sauce

2 tsp. Dijon

1 tbsp. tahini

1/2 tsp. paprika

Salt and pepper to taste

For pasta:

2-sweet potatoes

1-large mushroom cap

1 boneless chicken breast breast

Salt and pepper

Extra virgin olive oil

To Prepare:

Rinse the Quinoa with warm water and a dash of salt to remove the bitter outer coating.

Stir the quinoa while rinsing and use a fine mesh strainer. Shake the strainer to remove excess water before proceeding.

Bring water to a boil, add quinoa and simmer until all the liquid is absorbed.

Drain the excess liquid from the quinoa and fluff.

1. Use a spiralizer to transform the peeled sweet potatoes into noodle strip shapes. Chop chicken into small pieces.

2. Sauté the chicken in oil until brown on both sized. Salt and pepper each side lightly and remove from heat.

3. Sauté the mushrooms alone until they are tender. Put the chicken in with the mushrooms and sauté another 5 minutes. Add the sweet potato and cook until the sweet potato spirals are soft.

To Prepare Alfredo Sauce:

1. Mix all the ingredients for the Alfredo in a blender or food processor and mix on high until creamy.

2. Don't heat the sauce separately, but add it to the rest of the ingredients in the pan and heat.

Orchard Quinoa

You can almost imagine this being served as the midday meal in the South of Italy. Serve with a hearty red wine or strong lemonade for a perfectly refreshing meal.

You Will Need:

1 cup red quinoa

1/3 cup coconut oil

2 tbsp. red wine vinegar

1 1/2 tsp. shallots

Salt and pepper to taste

2 cups chopped tomato

1/2 cup chopped cucumber

3 tbsp. mint

1 tbsp. oregano

15 oz. can garbanzo beans

2 oz. feta cheese

Lemon wedges

To Prepare:

Rinse the Quinoa with warm water and a dash of salt to remove the bitter outer coating.

Stir the quinoa while rinsing and use a fine mesh strainer. Shake the strainer to remove excess water before proceeding.

Bring water to a boil, add quinoa and simmer until all the liquid is absorbed.

Drain the excess liquid from the quinoa and fluff.

1. Combine all the other ingredients together in a bowl, Mix well together and let chill for 1 hour.

2. Combine the quinoa with the mix. Serve with a topping of cheese and lemon wedges.

Zucchini Pasta with Vegan Meatballs

Here is a vegan twist on a classic Italian dish that you are sure to love. The quinoa makes the meatballs moister than the usual breadcrumb and flour fare, which makes it even better!

You Will Need:

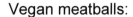

Vegan meatballs:

- 2 tbsp. coconut oil
- ½ medium onions
- 1 lb. small mushrooms
- 1 tsp. basil
- 1 tsp. parsley
- 1 tsp. oregano
- 1 tsp. chili flakes
- 1/2 cup sunflower seeds
- 15 oz. can lentils
- 1 cup quinoa
- 3 tbsp. quinoa flour

Zucchini Noodles:

- 3 zucchini
- 25-oz tomato sauce

To Prepare:

Rinse the Quinoa with warm water and a dash of salt to remove the bitter outer coating.

Stir the quinoa while rinsing and use a fine mesh strainer. Shake the strainer to remove excess water before proceeding.

Bring water to a boil, add quinoa and simmer until all the liquid is absorbed.

Drain the excess liquid from the quinoa and fluff.

1. Chop the mushrooms and onions. Preheat oven to 350.

2. Sauté onion and mushrooms until onions are clear. Add in the seasonings and stir well.

3. Pulse sunflower seeds in blender until coarse. Add sautéed ingredients to the blender along with ½ of the can of lentils and pulse until mixed.

4. Mix together with the remainder of the meatball ingredients in a bowl. Form into meatballs and bake on a sheet in the oven, turning once, until browned and crisp.

5. Cook and then cut the zucchini into spiralized spaghetti sized pieces.

6. Bring sauce to boil and then lower to simmer for 5 minutes. Serve over the zucchini with meatballs on top.

Spinach Quinoa with Tomato and Garlic

This is a light but warm meal to make that is perfect for removing the chill from the day. If you want, add a hearty sauce to it as well.

You Will Need:

1-garlic head

1 tbsp. coconut oil

1 tbsp. minced shallot

1/4 tsp. crushed pepper(red)

1/2 cup quinoa

1 tbsp. dry white cooking wine

1 cup chicken broth

1/2 cup baby spinach

1/3 cup diced tomato

1 tbsp. Parmesan cheese

salt

To Prepare:

Rinse the Quinoa with warm water and a dash of salt to remove the bitter outer coating.

Stir the quinoa while rinsing and use a fine mesh strainer. Shake the strainer to remove excess water before proceeding.

Bring water to a boil, add quinoa and simmer until all the liquid is absorbed.

Drain the excess liquid from the quinoa and fluff.

1. Wrap split and peeled garlic in baking foil and place in oven at 350 for about an hour. Remove the garlic. Let garlic cool. Mash the garlic to make the pulp.

2. Sauté shallots and pepper until the shallots are tender. Add in wine and broth, raise the temperature to a boil and then add in quinoa.

3. Reduce the temperature and simmer until all the liquid is absorbed.

4. Stir in the garlic and the remainder of the ingredients with a dash of salt and serve.

Conclusion

Thank you again for buying, "Quinoa: +25 Recipes For The World's Healthiest Super Food".

I hope this book was able to help you to discover the many ways that quinoa can be used in every recipe from anywhere in the world! You can understand now why quinoa is quickly replacing traditional rice and pasta in many dishes. It is flavorful, nutritious and easy to make.

The next step is to start experimenting with your favorite recipes to see how you can add more quinoa to your meals. This is also an important step towards better health, and a healthy lifestyle, for you and your family.

Finally, please take a couple of minutes and leave feedback and a review. My goal is to be a help so I take all feedback and apply it to my books. So if you loved the book or if you would have liked to see more added to the book please let me know. It'd be greatly appreciated!

Jessica

Printed in Great Britain
by Amazon